Put the Damn
Phone Down

Put the Damn Phone Down

Disconnect to Connect

ALYSSA LYNN MALMQUIST

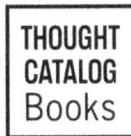

THOUGHT
CATALOG
Books

BROOKLYN, NY

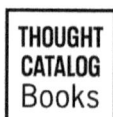

THOUGHT CATALOG Books

Copyright © 2018 by The Thought & Expression Co. All rights reserved.

Designed by KJ Parish.

Published by Thought Catalog Books, a publishing house owned by The Thought & Expression Co., Williamsburg, Brooklyn.

First edition, 2018

ISBN: 978-1-945796-97-5

Printed and bound in the United States.

10 9 8 7 6 5 4 3 2 1

*For **Josephine** and **Ralph**,*
who showed me limitless support, taught me endless life lessons,
and showered me with infinite love.
*For **Eileen** and **Hank**,*
who showed me authenticity, the importance of following your
passion, and how inner strength can help you overcome any
obstacle that comes your way.
I miss you all immeasurably.
I am forever grateful for your impact.

CONTENTS

Introduction

More content than ever before is being transported through our brains with the assistance of our devices. Unlimited amounts of information have become readily available to us whether it be on a phone, a computer, the television, or a tablet. As our focus has shifted to a digital realm, it is becoming more difficult for people to express their own thoughts or opinions.

We don't always have the chance to speak or the mindset to pull back as news is being thrown at us in all directions in every way possible.

This behavior is limiting our future generations as **we have more comparison and less freedom.**

Young people used to not care so much.

A time of experimentation, growth, and discovery is now documented, judged, and heavily examined.

The generation born into this digital age doesn't know a conversation or connection without the involvement of photographic evidence.

We have young people trying to rush through the initial stages of life, trying to emulate what they perceive as mature and beautiful. We're striving for what we believe to be happiness and accomplishment based on the social reality of others.

Older generations are trying to connect with younger generations, while younger generations are trying to

connect with strangers, while strangers are trying to connect with themselves.

As technology has made ginormous leaps, without pause, nearly all our communication is being replaced with devices.

Everything is digital:

Social Media. Phone calls. Texting. Advertising. Dating. E-Mail. Video. Shopping. Music. Banking. Photography. Gaming. Customer service. Interviewing. Meetings. Gambling. Research. Testing. Schooling.

The list goes on and continues to grow every day.

Suddenly, there are people that don't know how to connect without involving a phone or device. You see more people taking time to record everything just because they don't know how else to engage or spend their time.

The digital age has somewhat handicapped all humans, as our dependence has grown heavier on smartphone technology. Used as a preferential resource for communication, we're growing tired and lazy as our ambitions shrivel.

We're checking our phones for the sake of checking our phones. We aren't even thinking about it. We've become so attached to our devices that this behavior has morphed itself into a safety net.

We don't have to necessarily deal with the reality of situations in person anymore. If you're bored, you might text someone because of ease and accessibility. You may break up with someone over a text message simply because it's possible and easier than having to face it in person.

We send images in the forms of emojis and gifs without

actually saying anything. **We've limited our complex emotions into singular visuals.**

As great and temporarily hilarious as these visualizations may be, we've started entirely replacing words with them. In doing so, **we are no longer accessing that part of our brain that pushes us to form words and interact naturally.** Today, we don't even have to think. You can just snap a photo and send, in hopes of getting some sort of response.

The more we rely on technology to do the communicating for us, the more we cripple ourselves from communicating organically.

We've reached a point where we have abused the resources at our disposal, bleeding them dry as speed, accuracy, and accessibility have advanced beyond comprehension.

Maybe some of it was for the greater good, but I can't help but question if we progressed **too much too soon.** Have we progressed at a speed too fast for the human brain to process? **Are we so connected that we've become in fact disconnected?**

Are we really communicating anymore? Have we filled the void of deep and meaningful relationships with mindless, mediocre relationships? Have we become so reliant on technology and social media that we have begun to fear spontaneous communication? Are we drifting further and further away from authenticity?

In a world where we follow a surplus of people on a regular basis, are we no longer following ourselves? Have our own passions been pushed aside? Has our primary focus shifted to following a perception of people we idolize?

These are the questions that produce endless thoughts for me, taking up space in my mind, pushing me to share my thoughts with you and to dive into these topics in the following pages. I hope to push you to ask these same questions for yourself.

1

Social Media

In the late 90's, social media was born, and there was no turning back. Social media has become so accessible that we've reached a point of harmful interference with natural communication. I'm not claiming that all social media is bad. In fact, some of it can be very beneficial for businesses as well as people with long distance relationships between friends and family. But we live in a growing age of technology with **more changes than not**.

Social media allows anyone to amplify their perception to an unlimited audience. When social media evolved, individuals and businesses had an entirely different outlet to connect unlike ever before. As social media proved to increase a business's revenue, the term "influencer" was born as a new way for brands to connect with consumers. Influencers are people that use social media as a tool to make money while simultaneously making money for the brands that pay them.

As this phenomenon grew, so did the weight of that magic number of followers social profiles could attain. How many followers, along with the amount of engagement you have, determines an influencer's leverage in negotiating compensation within this type of transaction.

Now, everything has started to be treated like a business. First, we compete and compare to other social profiles. Then, we compete with our own content. What does best is what has the most likes. That contact can take place at that moment but also continue long thereafter. The ease of tracking engagement can become addictive. **How many likes and how many comments becomes a marker for success.**

With this behavior, we are no longer expressing ourselves for us. Our motivation for expression is sometimes entirely dependent on the need of reaction or attention from someone else.

There are two distinct types of social influencers. We have people who have already reached a level of fame that gain followers based off past work, whether it be a movie, television, music, fashion, sports, dancing, theater, business, etc. If they so choose, they can use social media to grow their following by posting frequently, engaging with followers, and collaborating with brands.

On the flip side, we have people that reach a level of fame **because of their social media profile.** They grow their following from content that followers are interested in. Maybe it's breathtaking views, or maybe it's nearly naked photos. Whatever the content is, it's enough to reel people in and keep them watching. Keeping people hooked takes **dedication, time, and consistency.**

I've noticed that many of these social media influencers who become relevant because of their social media status are posting at a compulsive rate. If they are doing something, it's being shared either live or in the form of photos and video.

Everything. Eating meals. Taking a walk. Driving. Waiting in line. Working out. Interacting with other people. Lying down. Playing with their animals. Doing their hair. Trying on clothes. **Everything.** Nothing is off limits. Even **doing nothing** is documented. Their focus intensifies on updating others while they aren't fully experiencing the updates themselves.

After recently moving to Los Angeles, I learned that *everyone* is a social media *star*. I use the term *everyone* lightly. Everyone's an *influencer* or a *public figure*. I learned that some people even buy followers. I repeat, you can buy social media followers. You can even buy likes. For some, it isn't necessarily about engagement anymore, but more about the number of people that follow you. Anything that can boost that ego or create the perception that we are at a higher level than others.

I had a branding company reach out to me about my Instagram when I first moved to Los Angeles. They found me after I started using the Los Angeles location marker on a few of my Instagram posts. Although uninterested, I was intrigued enough to hear what they had to say. I gave the guy I spoke with about four minutes before I hung up. He explained to me that my numbers weren't very good. He explained how my likes weren't doing so well on my last few posts and this was cause for distress. I played along and started explaining to him that he was the one reaching out to me and that I had no interest in purchasing any services from him.

His plan was to get me involved with his *influencer services* by bullying me into thinking that I needed more social acceptance. I verbalized my distaste in a **bold** manner.

He didn't like my reaction. He tried to manipulate me into thinking I needed a certain number of followers and likes to reach personal achievement and fulfillment in this "growing digital age." Although I was pretty sure I already knew the outcome, still I tried to open his mind to the idea that some people use social media merely to **express themselves creatively**. There are people that are satisfied without being social media *stars*. He continued to attack my Instagram profile and tried to push me into a way of thinking I was not interested in. So I ended up hanging up. But by playing along and having that debate, it really got me thinking.

Personally, I'm not interested in any of that. I think on some level we can all let our egos get the best of us. We like attention and feeling good about ourselves. Positive reinforcement is a nice feeling. That makes sense. But when we become so reliant on social acceptance and base our entire perception on the opinion of others, then we are hurting ourselves as we create barriers that limit our potential.

Social media *stars* or *influencers* have become so wrapped up in the attention to a level of excess. And it's never enough. We can track everything now: shares, likes, comments. It's all **updated by the second**, all from the people that **follow** us, as if **following** someone doesn't sound creepy enough.

We have people today that would absolutely crumble without social media. There are people that would not know what to do without the engagement and validation of others through digital technology and social media. I feel for the younger generations that know nothing else and were born into a time where the "social age" is all they know.

There are too many of us engaged with our devices, ignoring what's happening directly in front of us. **We are missing out on experiences and connections.**

Here is just one example that I am constantly reminded of:

When I see several people waiting at a crosswalk, disengaged and ignoring each other, I cannot help but wonder: What would happen if they didn't have their smartphones? Would they make a connection with someone they were meant to make a connection with? If they had made said connection, how would their lives be different? How much would that day change for them? Without making that connection, does that influence the rest of their lives?

Our hyper-focus on a digital universe is restraining our own firsthand experiences.

By putting so much of ourselves, our time, and our energy into devices, we miss out on true human connections we were meant to experience. Connecting with others allows us to feel on a deeper level.

As technology has progressed, we are under the impression that we are more connected than ever when the reality is the complete opposite.

It's all so **accessible**. So let's back up to where it all started: **smartphones.**

2

Smartphones

When's the last time you saw a restaurant give out crayons and paper to a child?

They don't need to anymore. The opportunity is rarely there because the accompanying adult has already placed some sort of digital device in front of them, leaving the child in a hypnotized zombie-like state. I cringe when I see a family out to dinner with their children connected to devices. **Literally, connected.** I've seen some kids fully strapped into devices, headphones and all, some so young that they haven't even learned to talk yet. How has it become so simple to make the decision to risk the initial stages of a child's development, with the goal of keeping them quiet for a specific period? We are hurting children in this case, while also limiting their capabilities when we think the solution to keeping them occupied is hypnotizing them with a smartphone or smart device. A concept so simple as crayons and sheet of paper that could allow a child to explore their creative eye, or express themselves through art, **replaced with a device.**

I think back to when I was in junior high and high school, circa 2005-2010. I remember how exciting it was when I got my first cell phone. It was a flip phone that could fit into the palm of my hand. I was limited to 100 text messages a month. So, if I was going to use a text, I had to make the most of each message. There was no time for one-word text messages, because that, would be **wasteful.** This was a time where wasting was a real concern. I had to make each text message count. My family also had a certain number of minutes a month that we could talk on the phone. So, it was the same with talking on the phone, **no wasting time**, more importantly **not wasting money.**

Fast forward to now where everything is **unlimited.**

We've reached a point where **being wasteful or excessive isn't even a concern.** I can't help but relate the **intake of digital content** to **food, drugs,** or **alcohol.** We are constantly monitoring calorie intake, and the food that enters our body. We've become more health conscious as well as more particular about what we put into our bodies. Same goes for alcohol. We have laws that limit us when it comes to operating a vehicle and even what age we must be to consume alcohol. Most drugs are prohibited by law, accompanied by extensive research on how negatively they can affect the brain.

But with our **smartphones and their applications**, we have **zero limits.** It doesn't matter the age or the amount of consumption you're taking on. There is **no limit. No laws are** regulating how often you use your smartphones. There is no measurement comparable to calorie intake that is broken down for you prior to smartphone use. We are using our devices without any limitations. I can't help but think what effect this is having on our mental health, not as clear and visible, as our physical health. So, because we aren't as focused on mental health, we don't see it as a problem.

By relying on computers and phones to do all the thinking for you, you begin to rely solely on devices, therefore ignoring your innate instincts. By not using your organic skills to communicate, you run the risk of losing them altogether.

We have smartphone applications that add filters and edit photos beyond reality... a reality only visible to the virtual eye. Now, we can communicate with someone **entirely** through a simulated reality. So, what happens to the generations that don't know a time before smartphones and social media? With every cause, there is an effect.

I know I'm generalizing, and this isn't the case for everyone. **However**, I can't help but be alarmed by the normality of excessive ego throughout social media today. You can create a perception of a lavish and seemingly perfect life. You can portray happiness even if it's not the case. You can angle your photos to create a body image of your choosing.

I think at the end of the day, a common goal for many is to ultimately be accepted by our peers. Social media allows you to update your audience as much as you'd like. The problem with that is that it makes it easier to obsess over the content we are updating.

Some can't function without having that smartphone in our hands. We rely on this device and at the very least, we need to know it's location, which cannot be physically too far away. It's always at arm's reach, and you see now more than ever, people **losing it** when they don't have that **crutch** of a phone to keep them from falling.

It feels good to talk to people but sometimes it can be scary. Whether it be an environment where we don't know anyone or an unfamiliar scene that just makes us feel uncomfortable, smartphones have become a reliable crutch to eliminate these feelings in certain situations. By not working through these feelings, we are jeopardizing our growth. No matter our external environment, we are dialed into this digital environment constantly. Instead of talking or even just accepting and experiencing solitude and silence, we often grab that smartphone and aimlessly scroll, allowing a surplus of content to enter past our corneas. Without thought, we've let so much information pass through our brains. Whether it's on a conscious level or not, it's **taking up space.** If you ask me, too much space. Space that has lasting effects on how we see ourselves and how we see other people.

We are harder on ourselves, and since we let so many people into our lives through social platforms, we are growingly preoccupied and concerned with how we look. Without thinking, based on the level of status a person seemingly has, we want to imitate that. We follow because we want to reach that level. We want to be the same.

There is too much simulated information running through our brains preventing spontaneous expression and natural thoughts. Our brains are clogged with endless information, most of which we don't need.

We see what's trending, and now more than ever, with the help of smartphone technology, we are trying to mirror it. We want to match what we see as the best. Just one example I've noticed on an extreme level is **appearance.**

3

Appearance

With the digital age, **beauty standards** have drastically changed.

The access to endless video tutorials alongside an oversupply of products and procedures has had a **hard** effect on the evolution of human appearance, women specifically. I think it's affected both genders, but more-so women. And as a woman, I can speak more to the impression on females.

Historically, we've judged women more critically than men. Let's be real: How often do we talk about the appearance of women? **Be honest.**

It's a lot. We talk about their:

- Hair type
- Hair color
- Hairstyle
- Too much makeup
- Not enough makeup
- Body build
- How skinny they are
- How skinny they aren't
- Length of legs

- Size of lips
- Shape of butt
- Skin clarity

And my personal favorite, **boobs.**

Let's talk about boobs for a second, the real kind more specifically. If a woman is blessed with big breasts, why is it that if there is any glimpse of cleavage, she's labeled negatively as promiscuous or scandalous? If another girl that happens to be flat-chested wears a top with a plunging neckline, but no cleavage exists, she's labeled positively sexy and confident.

We could have two women wearing the exact same top but **based on body type and size of body parts we judge who that woman is as a person.**

We judge women a lot.

- How many people they have slept with
- How many people they haven't slept with
- How successful they are
- How successful they aren't
- How emotional they are
- How emotional they aren't
- How strong they appear
- How weak they appear
- How much they ask for help
- When they don't ask for enough help

Not only are we judging physical attributes, but we build perceptions based on perceivable judgments. Where a man is passionate, a woman is crazy. Where a man is loving, a woman is too emotional. Where a man is strong, a woman is heartless. Where a man has opinions or thoughts, a woman is complaining or ranting.

Take my book for example. Some, without thinking, may associate my expression as an angry outburst because I am a woman. If I changed the author name to a man's name, my rant would probably be characterized as a perspective.

Conscious of that, I'm going to keep my female name on the cover.

Perhaps, again, I am generalizing but these **stereotypes** and perceptions are **still very real today**. In several styles of music, most strongly in rap and hip-hop, we are lowering the standards and potential of women.

If you have sex you're a **whore**. But be careful: If you don't have sex with anyone somethings wrong with you too. You're a **prude.** If you're not into a guy and turn them down you're a **bitch.** But again, if you are into them, don't take it too far. You run the risk of being called a **whore.** But you better do something; you wouldn't want to be labeled a **prude.**

I like to call this cycle the **cycle of stupid.**

Without using names, I can't help but compare musical artists that dive into heartbreak in their songs. Generally, if a man comes out with a song of heartbreak, we label him with positive attributes: loving, strong, deep, attractive, meaningful. Yet, if a female artist expresses heartbreak through just one song we label her with negative attributes: needy, attention-seeking, angry, weak, annoying. And of course, she can't complain about too many men, because women aren't supposed to share themselves with too many men. Whereas with men it's the complete opposite. Having a surplus of women at your disposal elevates you to a level of experience and power. You're the man. **This is where we are at** and I don't think enough attention can be brought to it right now.

So, let's circle back. This book isn't about gender inequality, but it **does** coincide with this topic of **appearance** I am dialing in on.

When we look at how much we hyper-focus on a woman's image and how intensely we are making judgments, it makes sense to me that some women have responded by severely altering their appearance. Alongside standards grown from social media and our digital world, plastic surgery and superficial enhancements have followed. Women are reacting and not in an encouraging way.

Surgery is becoming more normalized as we strive for an unrealistic expectation of perfection we view digitally. We want to get as close as we can to perfect as a result of comparing our own appearance to how others appear to us. We want to be accepted not only by men but by society.

Think of television and film. How often do you see a woman's naked body? And how many times do you see a man's naked body? I'm not saying there aren't naked men on film, but just compare how many times you've seen a penis to how many times you've seen nipples and vaginas.

Be honest.

Women are critiqued so heavily when it comes to appearance. If a guy isn't defined as handsome, he's able to outweigh that with money, a decent job, or even a comical personality. But if a girl isn't defined as physically beautiful, it's hard for people to move past that opinion onto anything else. **That's real, and it's anything but fair.**

I'm not sure when we made such a drastic shift, but accompanying the growth of social media and digital technology, we have shifted toward normalizing radical changes to our physical appearance.

Makeup and plastic surgery have advanced while becoming more accessible to a larger population. The new *beautiful* is being marketed as unreal, **literally.**

I think it's important to go through the awkward stages of puberty. When I was thirteen, I was in braces, wearing purple eyeshadow accompanied by chrome pink lipstick, and wearing padded bras. It was a troubling time, sure, but I got through it. More importantly, I grew, internally. It seems today, with the access to makeup tutorials and products, young people have perfected makeup application before they've even hit puberty. But even that wasn't enough.

Eyelash extensions and lip injections have become **common,** supplementing extreme contour and filled in eyebrows. Add filters and editing software, readily available for free, and we have girls of all ages trying to portray an idea of perfected beauty. **We are judging and limiting girls at a younger age than ever before.**

It's what we are perceiving from mindless reality stars that we've elevated to a status of following. We have so many in the limelight sending a message of what beautiful can be with the help of digital and physical alterations. Idolizing these perceptions has given more power to them while taking away personal power from ourselves.

It used to be hairy vaginas and hard nipples. Now it's fake

lips, fake hair, fake boobs, fake eyelashes, and colored contacts. We've altered our most natural self. **And for what?**

These models or influencers that try to deceive you into a perception of perfection aren't helping. I'm not saying there isn't beauty in modeling or photography. But when we create an image that only allows people to see us as perfected, edited, and enhanced, that is **not real.**

And sure, the concept may seem simple as I'm spelling it out, but it's not being practiced if we're buying these products these influencers promote, watching them on mindless reality television, or comparing our lives to what they portray digitally.

When we ignore our most natural selves, we raise this perception by reacting and trying to replicate it. We are losing what makes us unique and becoming more alike.

Acne is real. Scars are real. Bodies are real. Imperfections are real. They differentiate us from others and define us as individuals. They make us uniquely unique.

Genuineness is diminishing as we boost the ego of some, instantaneously **lowering the self-esteem of others.**

As a result, I believe we are comparing ourselves to others more intensely and regularly. Comparing ourselves to seeming perfection can have a negative influence on how we see ourselves. I think there is a direct link to this behavior and the changes we've seen in recent years with self-esteem, anxiety, and depression.

4

Mental Health

According to the National Center for Health Statistics, "Suicide rates among teenage girls between the ages of 15 and 19 are at an all-time high in the last 40 years. Suicide rates doubled among teenage girls and grew by more than 30 percent for teenage boys in this age group between 2007 and 2015."

So is there a link between the increase in suicide and the increase is social media? I'm not going to dive in too deep with facts and statistics but based on observation and instinct; **I believe there is.** I can only share my stance on the topic based on observation, common sense, and intuition. I encourage you to think for yourself and decide for yourself. But don't ignore the reality we're currently a part of.

Depression is growing, right alongside suicide at a time where we are comparing ourselves to others at a more powerful pace than ever before. Suicide has increased overall for both genders, and I can't help but think that this tragic reality is the outcome of constant comparison to ourselves with people we connect with digitally. We are in a relentless competition for more attention, more likes, more engagement. **Success is**

measured on followers and likes, two actions that take little to no effort.

Relinquishing power to a perceived digital world can inflict insecurities, self-doubt, and unnecessary sadness. And without limiting or monitoring our intake of potentially toxic realities, we are scarring ourselves without comprehension. We're giving a lot of power away when we ignore our intuition, and what we believe to be beautiful, expressive, or happy.

Common sense is dwindling. We're living during a time of constant noise that doesn't ever shut down. We've started weakening our minds by ignoring the parts of the brain that produce real and natural thoughts or opinions. Power has been assigned to what digital limitations tell us what things should look like. The comparison is lowering our confidence based on what we perceive others to have.

I can't help but push those relinquishing their self-power to understand the concept of those pushing perfection and unreal beauty through social platforms: They depend on you for validation, but their power is created by lowering the self-esteem of others. It's **ugly.**

Their resources are limitless. Money is a large factor in making nearly everything possible today. Makeup artists, hair stylists, expensive and extensive products, photographers, image-editing software, and so much more.

And for social media stars that would like you to believe they are leading lives full of constant beauty, perfection, or true happiness, it's not always going to be the case. It's almost always not going to be the case. No one's lives are perfect. We know this. There's good and bad for all of us. That's how the balance works in life. We all have highs and we all have lows. It's how we react to the lows that shape us into who we are.

The most genuine forms of happiness are created from moments only shared with a limited number of people. Maybe it's in a relationship, friendship, or shared with your family. But the distinct details aren't shared with a surplus of strangers. **Opening your life up to a limitless number of people who follow you lessens the impact of your memories or experiences, no matter how perfect the digital world may make them seem.**

And the harsh reality is that most of these social media influencers aren't allowing you into their lives for the primary goal of connection. The target is **idolization, riches, and status.**

Ignore what others appear to have in the digital realm. Focus more on what you do have in your reality and on your own personal journey.

When comparing yourself to other people becomes adapted into your routine it turns into regular behavior. However, in doing so, you carry this **needless weight** of information with you into whatever else you're doing. This could result in feelings of overwhelming sadness because we start to feel that we don't have what we think someone else does.

The reality is, a lot of it is **not real.**

Filters. Angles. Edits. Surgical enhancements. Painted faces. Perfect body shape. Exaggerated body parts.

It's a perception, an altered perception. And I'm not saying it's all bad. But I think the bad is becoming more and more normalized and we're losing authenticity. As we lose authenticity, we open ourselves up to insecurities.

You know what's beautiful?

- Originality
- Authenticity

- Open-mindedness
- Acceptance
- Connection
- Selflessness
- Inspiration
- Creation
- Love

With a detailed focus on a digital world, we're losing what's most naturally beautiful at our core both physically and intellectually.

It's becoming more difficult to communicate purely. We still want natural and genuine connection when what we're putting in is grossly unnatural. We live in a time where so many are accessible to us, even those we probably should have let go of, for the sake of our sanity.

Whether it be someone you were in a relationship with or even a past friend, they aren't in your life for a reason. So why do so many of us keep track the social media postings of people who are no longer in our lives? We're driving ourselves mad focusing on the irrelevant details of people who are we are no longer in physical contact with.

We don't need to know who our exes are spending time with. We don't need to know what people who've hurt us are doing. Even for people who haven't hurt us, we don't need to know what they're doing, either. But most importantly, we don't need to stay connected with people we are trying to move on from or who have already left our lives.

Moving on is incredibly difficult, and the digital world has pushed us to believe that we don't have to disconnect from anyone. Seemingly staying connected is more comforting than the alternative, but I can't help but wonder what effect that has on the mind.

We aren't thinking of what is better for our mental health in the long run. We are only concerned with comforting ourselves in the present by not letting go and holding on to whatever we can from our past. I think this has hurt us today and it's getting worse as we share so much of our lives through a social world. It's all too much.

We are meant to meet and connect with certain people throughout our lives. Some are meant for particular stages while others stay with us for longer periods of time throughout our lives. With the assistance of social media and digital technology, we aren't really letting go of anything or anyone anymore. Our present is being affected because we're still somewhat connected from the past.

Not only do we want to know any and all information about people from our past, we want to know all of this information about people that could be a part of our future; people we haven't even had the chance to meet yet. Cue **dating applications.**

5

Dating Applications

Relying on social networks and smartphone applications to stay in constant contact with others has completely affected how we meet new people and how we look for relationships. When it comes to wanting a relationship, we don't have to communicate in person anymore. We don't have to communicate in person at all if we don't want to. It can all be virtual. We can make multiple selections and talk with multiple people at once. We swipe, and we judge others based on an intentionally selected photo and an unverified biography. Our expectations have grown because of how we perceive a virtual reality.

We want genuine relationships that match up with our expectation of what we think our happiness should look like. We want that genuine connection while putting in the exact opposite amount of disingenuous effort.

We judge people solely based on photographs and detailed explanations of their past experiences and future aspirations. This is how we choose to determine who we allow the opportunity to engage in a forced interaction with us.

When did we become so high-maintenance? Our minimal

bare standards have shifted toward knowing a person's entire background, their habits, how they photograph, and their views before we can even consider giving them the opportunity to have a chance to meet us.

When did that stop being the exciting stuff you discover throughout a relationship?

And on the receiving end, when did we did we become so self-obsessed with making sure we all at least portray the image that we are all living the most exaggerated version of lives?

We are striving for an unrealistic and altered vision of perfect because of our environment, while we perceive information from the digital world.

But this is where we're at. **Today we have apps.**

To speak accurately about them, I downloaded two of these dating applications. I thought, "I can't talk about dating applications if I didn't at least do my research and have all the necessary information."

I wanted to see what all the fuss was about and be able to truthfully say that at least I tried it. So I downloaded these apps onto my phone, two of several dating applications readily available to people of all ages, at no monetary cost. But is there **a cost**…?

We can download these apps and immediately have a surplus of options. We are presented with a planned perception someone has chosen to be their first impression. You're able to plan what you say and how you look. You can create whatever perception you want, whether it's true or not. You can talk to as many people as you'd like all at once. Your options are **unlimited.** Cue the start of the **hookup generation.** It works for some people, depending on where they're at with their experience. Although the casual thing can work for a while and with certain people, it can be exhaustingly unfulfilling.

We've made quite the drastic change from the generations before us. People used to get married much younger and sometimes never had the chance to explore other options. Now we have too many options available to us and we're losing the capabilities to interact spontaneously and unplanned. We're afraid more than ever to choose someone, knowing how accessible and endless our other choices can be.

Dating has morphed into a hot mess and being the old soul that I am, I can't help but crave something of more substance and truth.

With the increase in options, so much communication has become forced and unnatural. Why wouldn't it? We don't *need* to put in the effort anymore. It's all been simplified and increased in speed. Because there is a lack of effort, there is a lack of commitment and everything has become much more casual.

With so many options at our fingertips, if there is something minor that turns us off, we move on to the next. We've become pickier. We can always find another option with little to no effort. With a surplus of options, I think our attention span has diminished, creating a rarity in authentic relationships. You don't have to be in a relationship to have sex. You don't need to have an emotional connection with someone to be intimate.

Our relationships are coming and going at a growing pace. We are constantly hooking up without the exclusivity. If you want someone else, or an additional someone else, you can find that with the click of a button. By making it a habit, you can build upon deeper issues from relationship to relationship without even realizing it.

There are always going to be more options. **Too many options, if you ask me.** I think the excess of options has led us to overthink about what is going on right in front of us. I think it's driven us to destroy relationships that made us happy for the hope that there is bigger and better, even if what we already have is big and great. **Have our expectations become so unrealistic because so much of what is seemingly bigger and better isn't real?**

Are we setting expectations that can never be met while sabotaging the relationships in front of us? Moving at such a rapid pace, we may not always be taking the time to decipher what is happening here and now. And I think to an extent, we're missing out.

We can't expect natural and genuine relationships when we are spending so much of our time dialed into the screens on our devices, making visual judgments on anyone and anything we happen to scroll by. We can't become these egomaniacs that have become so self-obsessed with dating profiles and social accounts that we start pushing away people that don't meet our delusional standards. We all deserve happiness and to experience real human connection in many forms, but **we can't continue on this path of ever-growing superficiality.**

If we want more, we must do more. You give what you get, and a little effort goes much further thank you think.

The same goes for business. We can't expect long-term and substantial growth if you're only putting in short-term and minimal commitment. But **brands have gotten lazy.** We used to have limited celebrity promotions, but now in a social world, we've extended that to a much larger group of unlimited *influencers.*

6

Branding

When did brands get so lazy? Coming from a background in marketing, I can't help observing as I try to determine when exactly brands decided to use anyone and anything to promote their products. I can't help but wonder when the turning point occurred where businesses decided to rely so heavily on the chance that a random influencer could sell their products for them. From a financial standpoint, it totally makes sense. **For the now.** Having an influencer post on your behalf through social media can ignite consumer attention in a fast and simplified manner. This can be followed by a sequential bump in sales and revenue. But in terms of long-term profit, loyalty, and credibility, this tactic lacks substance.

Paying someone a large amount of money just to promote a product on their social media should offend consumers. Brands are banking on the fact that you'll associate the admiration of your favorite celebrity and/or influencer and that it will translate and copy over to trust and a new admiration of the brand or product. **Brands are banking on the fact that you don't have the capacity to think for yourself** in hopes that you will act without contemplation.

Influencers don't care if your teeth are whitened or your hair has volume. Influencers aren't concerned with how fake your lips look or what products you can contour your face to create an illusion. Influencers aren't passionate about what tea you're drinking. Influencers don't care about how you'll be affected by their promotion. Influencers are invested in how many people they can convince to use their code, which will determine their financial payout.

I think at first product promotions made sense. Initially, products were paired with people in a scenario where the product matched the promotion. We then got to a place rooted in greed and laziness, to where we're pairing products onto influencers that have no relationship or anything in common with the product or brand whatsoever.

This transaction isn't benefiting anyone but the people on the receiving end of the payout. We aren't necessarily using people of status or accomplishment anymore: it's more about that magic follower number. A number that's losing validity by the day as so many have attempted to cheat their way to perceptual stardom by purchasing fake followers.

There are still some with credible followings that produce engagement. This group consists mainly of people who were lucky enough to hit social media status at that block of time when social media started blowing up. It was a few years after social media had been around: right before we made that giant dive into social over reality.

A number of people who have reached a prominent level of following owe their success to right place right time. *Fame* has become more attainable and quicker to achieve. Having so many people who are accessible and reachable didn't necessarily take time or effort to get to a level of recognition.

Being at the start of this trend placed people at the forefront of this follower trend. This set influencers up to piggyback their successes while remaining relevant and gaining more promotional offers.

It's unfortunate that the more common as this has become, most of us are no longer allowing ourselves to think. It's troubling to think we are **no longer forming our own opinion** on brands and products as we choose to take the word of an influencer, as long as whoever is attached to the promotion means enough to us at that temporary moment in time. With so much noise coming at us, our own thoughts are being ignored and we are relying on whoever makes their way onto our phone or computer screen.

Reality stars and Instagram models rely on this thought process as a means of income and financial stability. It's gotten so out of control, it's growing more common while more and more people are striving to be in a position where they can make money for posting one photo on their Instagram.

The payout doesn't even come close to measuring out the work put in. There are average people making yearly salaries from long hours and constant effort that may work an entire year just to make what an influencer can make by posting three photos. **I'm not promoting one extreme or the other, but it's hard to grasp how exactly this shift in society is going to affect us going forward.**

People have become strictly invested in creating a personal brand, treating themselves and their influence as a business. Although this may be valid in some cases of people that reach a certain level of experience and attainment, there are so many that have sunk into self-obsession that we're living in a world where delusional self-publicists are digitally making their way into our lives via smartphones and social media.

I acknowledge that we are in a state of progression, and of course, things are naturally going to change. **And they should.** But the direction brands have taken in shoving product to consumers is just a mindless way of making little effort and commitment while hoping for a big payout.

Just because we saw someone on our favorite reality television show doesn't mean they know what vitamins we should be taking. Just because we idolize someone based on looks doesn't mean we need to be buying their makeup line because they had the unlimited resources to pay a team to do all the work, and then decided to attach their name at the end with no risk or effort. And just because someone just so happens to have over 20,000 followers on Instagram, it doesn't mean we need to buy the face cream they have decided to overpoweringly, and most likely insincerely, promote.

And hey, maybe it some situations the promotion is true and sincere, and that's great. But the point I am really trying to drive here is, **why are we so trusting in the opinions of others when we are perfectly capable** of making decisions ourselves?

Why can't products rely on the quality of their product? Why are brands choosing to force an attachment to products with someone that has nothing to do with the product or business?

More importantly, **why are we so aimlessly trusting in people we don't actually know to make decisions for us that involve health, beauty, food, and so on?**

Is it because our progression in social media and technological quality has pushed us to the point where we feel as though we do *know* these people? And because we do *know* these people, should we trust that their needs will fit and match ours based on our perception of them that seemingly relates us?

We need to take a step back. We need to realize we aren't truly connected to everyone, although social media tricks us into thinking otherwise. Not only has this been relevant to business, but it's also traveled over into the world of media. The world of casting has changed when it comes to television and movies. Casting roles aren't always done in person as it was in the past. It's done virtually. It's sought out through social media platforms for people that appear to be the real deal.

So, what happens when you have someone on social media that is so theatrical, so animated, so entertaining, but then you take them outside of their comfort zone into unfamiliar territory? What happens when you put them in front of a real camera and they don't perform the same way?

What happens when you put someone in a situation where the communication is happening in real time in person, and that's not something they're used to?

7

Acting

Temporary success in one area can last long-term in other areas. Today, by attaining a significant amount of social media followers based on one successful project, you can finalize job opportunities for you in the future.

You don't even have to work anymore, not continuously anyways. This may not be the case for everyone, but it is in fact for some. You may not even need to create updated content. Things are becoming less unique and more repetitive. Do one thing to get noticed enough and you can ride that train for as long as you want, dependent on your social media following of course. It doesn't matter if you're talented or if you bring the most creativity to the project, it's about how many people you can get onboard from your following. And a lot of it is relentlessly mindless.

As a writer and actress in Los Angeles, I can't tell you how many castings I've seen that have made a high social media following into a prerequisite to an audition. Coming from **Massachusetts**, this was a huge culture shock for me. Many people I've met in Los Angeles have already jumped on this current trend of buying social followings and forcing content out that presents them in an untrue light.

You're competing with legitimate and illegitimate competition. The two are intertwined and it's becoming more difficult to tell which is which.

As a creative, I can't tell you how much I struggle with loving the creative outlet that is social media while also observing how detrimental it's been in the creative process. I want to create. I want to write. I want to express myself.

We have people in the music, film, and television industry that have been tricked into thinking social media is the determinant of whether their creations will bear success.

Actors are buying social media followers in hopes of landing more auditions. Creative projects are creating social accounts to document and share every minuscule detail from start to finish. It's no longer about putting all your effort into the vision and final project. Creatives are restricted in updating followers with appropriate and strategic content to establish continued relevance. We aren't necessarily creating to create anymore. It's about establishing your brand, repeatedly updating your following, and making a constant effort to remain relevant.

And why? For what?

In the same way, your followers really shouldn't care what you're doing every second of the day, and you shouldn't care about the number of people that are obsessing over you. Who cares about likes or views; some are bought, most are mindless. Why have we been deceived into thinking that this signifies importance? The number of people following you has nothing to do with the creative process and what you're able to produce.

You're just aligning yourself with **reality stars** that are posting perfected and professional photos of their seemingly perfect lives. You're regrouping yourself into a pool of **YouTubers** that have attained fame by updating people with what they're doing from sunup to sundown. You're matching the neurotic effort at perfecting a theme for **social bloggers** that push an abundance of useless products accompanied by planned testimonials.

There's too much noise, too much distraction. And those distractions allow people without talent to rise without internal growth. Creative roles are distributed based on social media following without looking at actual talent. So there are people that quite possibly were meant for roles being denied wrongly, creating a heavy imbalance of garbage we see on screen today.

I can't help but think of reality stars turned authors or influencers. I can't help but think of influencers turned health experts or actors. I can't help but think of actors or **reality stars turned politicians**. This has created a giant shift in power when it comes to **certain people who have wrongfully been placed in roles of leadership**.

Credibility seems to be a thing of the past. Experience can be promoted even if it's disingenuous. Some of it's credible, but a lot of it is garbage. The lines are blurry, as anyone with enough of a following can produce a show, film, book, or any creative project by simply attaching their name.

Power is perceived more heavily today entirely based on the size of your "following," and social media has allowed people to follow a limitless amount of people.

You don't need to be a creative to create. **I'm not saying that certain people shouldn't create. I believe we're all capable of creating.** But there's a process. There is time and effort.

There is reflection and thought. It's not mindless and slapped together.

I believe there are still several talented people who have risen to a level of achievement today. **But** there are plenty of people without talent who also have attained a similar status and united themselves to a level of misconception. In certain scenarios, people without experience or talent have ascended through the creative pipeline based on social following. It translates not only in television in film but also in music.

Today it just takes a certain number of followers to star in a music video and suddenly go on tour. You don't even need to sing. Your voice can be changed, and your performance can be edited. Vocal range, performance skill, and true talent are no longer essentials.

As a result, we've had a lot of crap pass through our brains. It's loud and it's relentless. It makes it harder to determine what exactly we are taking in.

Sure, we can watch reality stars as they are putting on makeup, live and in real time. We can watch YouTube stars as they are eating breakfast. We can watch Instagram influencers visit a resort on a paid promotional vacation. The camera never stops rolling. At the end of the day, the only thing that ultimately matters is how much money can be made. **Money.** It makes sense, although no amount is ever enough. And with money comes power, and with power comes ego.

By idolizing people with the means and resources of creating perfected visual perceptions of reality we can become locked into these misconceptions and drag them into our daily lives and views. We can translate these perceptions into our own realities.

But by following, watching, and engaging, we are

simultaneously elevating some to a higher power. As the self-esteem lowers for many, **the ego of few is in continuous escalation.** By taking part and engaging in monotonous and constant content, we are feeding the **ego** of people who believe they need to be worshiped and followed.

8

Ego

Although many of us would find it hard to admit, we've all made a ginormous shift when it comes to ego. Social media gives people the platform to express themselves in whichever way they choose. You're able to throw out your opinions and/ or complaints with a visual megaphone.

But when did everyone start to think that everyone cares about what you think? Or what one does? Or what one eats? Or what one suddenly feels? Or what one wants to complain about?

Aggressive as it may be, I truly wonder when we started to believe that people cared so much about constant and repetitive updates from our daily routines all the way to political viewpoints?

Facebook has turned into a one-sided therapy session. Sometimes people engage, and you have these big topics and conversations being dissected through computers and phones with no real-life engagement. Instagram has tricked us into thinking everyone's a model or a brand influencer.

Most people are under the delusional impression that they have an audience that cares about the trivial details that make up their everyday lives; it's terrifying. We're so preoccupied with updating people on restaurants we're eating at or shows we're watching and who we're doing these activities with. We are distracted by updating others that we are nowhere close to being fully present, missing out on the full experience of what we're doing and who we're doing it with. If we aren't writing out an update, we're streaming it by video and photos. I've become horrified by the common scene when I'm out and every single person has their phone pointed on a shared focal point, as each person modifies their perception and makes the choice to watch through their lenses. Almost no one is ever watching with their eyes. The top priority is to make sure that everyone else sees and is hopefully jealously impressed.

Mystery is fading away. Some things are meant to be kept private.

The ego is intensifying visually as our worth is being determined by the engagement of the content we post. How many likes, how many comments, and how much money we can make off our look.

I think there's a big misconception of women who claim to promote positivity and beauty while only pushing out altered content that places them in a position of status or power. Positivity is not putting others down, **intentionally or not**, to make yourself feel more empowered.

Beauty isn't an insatiable need for attention. Beauty isn't longing for idolization. Beauty is not pumping your ego daily and evaluating said beauty on the engagement you're getting from a digital platform. Beauty isn't strategically pushing people to become invested with you from a digital distance. Beauty is not posting pictures where your face is edited, your poses are forced, and your imperfections are erased. Beauty is not posting the same photo of yourself daily with a different backdrop in hopes of others worshipping you.

We all have imperfections and they are not only beautiful, they're real.

We need to embrace our natural selves and flaws now more than ever. Sure, maybe sometimes you aren't natural but it's all about balance. It's when you're portraying this image of flawlessness and the incapability of blemish that you're hurting other people. We have seemingly perfect bodies, mostly all retouched, flooding our social devices today. Certain angles, filters, and editing skills have created an illusion that this is what we should strive for in real life.

I want to be clear: my intention is not to put down women who are revealing or promiscuous. **Who cares about how many clothes you are or aren't wearing.**

But, a girl taking her clothes off for social validation has become overwhelmingly and grossly common. It's constantly flooding the social world because certain women have promoted this idea that if you reveal enough of your body it will bring you status, followers, and the financial payout of your dreams. That greed gets seen and shines through on these photos.

No one's life is perfect, not even for a second. What matters is what you're comfortable with. What matters is being authentic and real. And I think it's clear that a lot of women aren't comfortable with what they're putting out there because you can tell when it's unnatural.

But we care less about what we're comfortable with and more about boosting our own ego to the point that it becomes uncontrollable.

So when exactly was the turning point when we became **a generation of self-obsessed egomaniacs?**

Digital technology has given us an outlet to create and express but so often has been abused and taken advantage of by the ever-growing egos of today. It's **gross.**

Not only do we feel the need to constantly promote and boost our own personal ego, but that also translates into the ego of our relationships. We entice people to get invested into our relationships when we are constantly posting intimate and dramatic professions of our love. Couples are competing with couples.

- Who has the better looking significant other
- Who has the better love story
- Who travels the most
- Who loves each other the most
- Who's strongest together
- Who's happier together
- Who has the better family
- Who has the best kids
- Who has the best pets
- Who has the best anniversary celebration
- Who has the best Valentine's celebration
- Who goes on the best honeymoon

We are all guilty of this on some level. Weddings are competing with weddings. Newborns are competing with newborns. The same goes for gender reveals, birthday parties, vacations, engagements, workouts, body image, diet, meal prep, fashion, etc. These big moments are becoming less about self-discovery and expression and more about competition.

We've been pushed into thinking we need to express our

most heartfelt emotions through social media posts and that those posts give the relationship validation.

Our most heartfelt expressions are becoming reusable and losing their sincerity. I think it's fine to express whatever it is you want to express on whichever outlet you choose, but when that doesn't translate in person is where it gets concerning. When you think that expressing a birthday sentiment or congratulations through social media but never bother to express that through talking over the phone or in person, you're minimizing the genuineness. You're replacing in-person communication with a digital supplement.

It becomes less about the person you're writing about and more about how others will perceive your deepest expressions. Celebrities do this a lot on social media. They think millions of people need to know about the most intimate details about their anniversaries, children, parties, vacations, meals, adventures, etc. They believe their millions of followers need to know that they still love their significant other and how much they love them. They think we need to know what their infant children look like days out of the hospital. They think we need to know it all. With this behavior, "celebrity" or not, we're expressing sentiments motivated by outside judgment. We're oversharing in competition and finding it easier to do online versus in person. But the more detail we share the more we minimalize the meaning of our words.

The more we focus on our own ego, the less confident we become. There's a distinct difference between confidence and ego. **Confidence is quiet; ego is loud.**

When you celebrate yourself and express yourself creatively, it's about you and for you. **It's beautiful.**

When you pump your own ego only to elevate yourself

above others, you believe that you deserve a status of elevation. **It's ugly.**

The cost of achievement shouldn't be the defeat of others.

It's not just toxic for the people that are ingesting the constant ego, but it can also be detrimental to the *celebrity or influencer.* In certain instances, an influencer may not always end up receiving the engagement they wanted or expected, pushing them to ironically also obsess and overthink. It's a lethal cycle. Insecurity and self-doubt can find their way traveling back onto you. **Relying on others to feed your own ego also gives them the power to starve your ego.**

So for those of you that believe your social media status determines who you are, ask yourself: Is the cost of focusing so much on the opinions of others for potential power worth not following your own true passions? And please don't try to say that your passion is being famous or worshipped. That's not passion; that's nauseating.

It's great to engage with the people you care about and know. But it's really not okay to have that same level of engagement with **strangers**: people you've never actually met. This puts fault onto both sides of the problem.

We need to get past this idea of this ever-growing common goal of having a high number of strangers can validate what we're doing. Break the spell and stop thinking that being an influencer is your destination to fulfillment and achievement because it's not. That greed will lead you to a place of loneliness and emptiness where evolvement or change do not exist.

The only person you should be following is **yourself.**

9

Follow Yourself

I'm not saying all social media is bad. I'm not saying that time should have stood still without progression; of course not. But we're at a point where real-life communication is frequently being replaced with social messages, text messages, dating applications, and the growing forms of technological communication.

We can't expect texts and emojis to translate our emotions. True emotion can have several facets. There can be more than one emotion in a feeling or an expression.

We've become so focused on how exciting and adventurous another person's life can be while abandoning attention to our own lives, our own passions, and our own path. And the intensity of this shift is having a drastic effect on how we perceive ourselves and each other. When we utilize technology to do all the communicating for us, we are losing the ability to connect with one another in real time. And the **ability to connect with one another is one of the greatest feelings we can experience** with another human being.

It all goes back to human connection. **Everything. All of it.** It's what we all, as humans, crave and desire. We want to feel a connection to others and experience mutual feelings of reciprocated connection. We want to feel love, friendship, and companionship. We want to feel passion, excitement, and adventure.

Digital technology has tricked us into thinking we are able to stay connected with everyone now. At times we are so connected that we feel we are a part of the pregnancy, vacation, or graduation as nothing is kept private. We're sharing everything and anything for attention, engagement, and reassurance. There isn't an end to any of it. But the harsh reality is, that is not how life works.

Things do come to an end.

Relationships come to an end. Experiences come to an end. Lives come to an end.

It's sad but beautiful. Awful then exciting. Terrible but hopeful. **New relationships start. New experiences unfold. New lives begin.**

So are we fully able to accept new when we're still so involved with the past? Or are we desperately trying to hold on to so many average relationships that we can't fully accept authentic relationships nor nourish our most important relationship: **the relationship we have with ourselves?**

Different people have different impacts on us throughout our lives. It can be as small as a smile from a stranger that turns our entire day around. It can be as big as a role model that has a true influence on the person we grow to be. I hate to use the terms "role model" and "influence," as these words have taken on entirely new meanings today. But, there are still people who can have an authentic and genuine interest in being there with you and for you during the growing stages of your lives. I was lucky enough to have some amazing influences growing up, some with me still and some not. But what's truly amazing is when an impact can live beyond a person's lifespan. I am lucky enough to know what that feels like. But because I am lucky enough to know what that feels like, I can't help but want that for everyone else.

Quality over quantity.

We aren't necessarily meant to hang on to everyone throughout our lifespan. As temporarily sad as it may be, it's beautiful to move on, evolve, and allow new people into your life. We aren't meant to stay perceivably connected with every single person we encounter. It feels good to stay connected. It feels better than the alternative, which is saying goodbye without knowing if or when we'll see that other person again.

Maybe it's someone we loved on a television show. Or maybe it's someone we met at a party that we got along with and had an enjoyable conversation. Maybe it's a current significant other's family member. Maybe it's an ex-relationship. Maybe it's an old boss at a job we left. Maybe it's a teacher that inspired us in a way we never knew. Maybe it's a coworker that made a hard job easier. **Maybe.** Relationships that ended good, bad and everything in between are being followed through a digital world. There are endless people we're interacting with throughout our lives, and sometimes you need to just take those interactions for what they are.

We are constantly making connections with the people in front of us and at a distance. But latching on and staying connected to every single person's journey through a digital eye is an overload of information that has a direct effect on our own journey.

Whether it be romance, friendship, or family, **our relationships determine who we are.** We are a result of how we treat ourselves and how we treat others. When we lose the authenticity of those connections, we lose ourselves. **Always do you.**

I challenge you to **disconnect** in a world that's so connected. This may be the way society has shaped itself today, but you are in full control of your actions. Don't think of it like you're missing out. Think of it like **you're finally not missing out.**

Put forth a conscious effort to experience what's going on around you. Go out with your friends and be fully present. Put the phone away. Make a conscious decision to limit the time spent disconnected from reality and connect with what's happening in the real world. Go up to someone and start a conversation. Be okay with silence and reflection. **Nourish your mind with organic human contact.**

Take some time to yourself and **put the damn phone down.** Get off your social media accounts for a few days. You can even designate one day a week that you don't touch your social media. You don't need to delete your profiles but delete the apps from your phone. Notice the number of times you go to check social media on your phone without thinking and remembering they aren't on your phone. **Take note of how many times you forget.**

When these platforms of fabricated communication are so easily accessible, it can become addictive, habitual, and built into our daily routines.

Without the distraction of constant social media updates, you have the chance to realize who you are truly communicating with. Observe who is making an effort and who you have decided to make an effort for.

Surrounded by chaos and uncertainty, **one thing you will always have control over is yourself and the choices you make.**

Be fully present in a world that makes it easy not to be. **Be you for you.**

When you follow yourself, you can tap into the infinite number of ways you can **express yourself.**

10

Express Yourself

It's time to shift the focus back on ourselves. We can allow the technological world to be a part of our lives, but we cannot allow it to be our entire lives. Social boundaries are limiting our expression. **We're losing authentic relationships while obsessing over the lives of others.** Others are obsessing over sharing their lives and every detail that follows.

If something truly awesome is happening in front of you, experience it. You don't need to document it alongside a sea of other phones documenting the exact same moment. Be the **only one** watching without the limitation of a technological device. My hope, eventually, is that you may not be the **only one**.

I don't want any of us to miss out, and right now, that's exactly what we're doing. We're missing out on memories. We are so preoccupied with having the memories locked and recorded into these devices that **we're ignoring the first and only chance we have to fully experience our memories.** We aren't even using this part of our brains anymore. We're **dependent on these devices to handle the memory storage for us.**

At a time where issues are seemingly being projected and discussed more than ever, don't abuse technological advances for your own personal motives. Using words or slogans that align with trends and popularity doesn't always mean the person is being true to themselves. Social technology gives anyone and everyone a platform, whether they know what they're talking about or not.

Just like social media, the news can be tweaked, too. We've got a whole lot of stupid coming at us right now as we have a microscope on all that is happening in the world, accompanied by the resources to alter.

The words "fame" and "idol" are used so commonly as we raise so many onto a pedestal. And this limelight has stolen so many into a state of greed and dependence.

People have become addicted to digital tricks that allow them to be promoted as perfected states of being. People have gotten carried away with perfecting angles, editing, and enhancements.

Recognize the level of superficiality that runs through this cycle.

Outlets used to express creativity and originality have been misused and abused into creating false realities free of flaws and error.

We think the abundance of information out there gives us endless knowledge. We're comparing our lives and our problems to the lives and problems of others. **The internet gives us so many answers leading us to believe there is an answer to everything.** We think we can search for any problem on the internet, making us all doctors, therapists, and experts.

Feeling anxious isn't anxiety. Feeling sad isn't depression. Feeling crazy isn't crazy.

Too much information is at our fingertips, making us impatient and misleading us to believe we know more than we do. In actuality I think we may know too much; too much to determine what is accurate and what isn't.

We ingest all this information thinking we know it all, ignoring instinct and common sense. You can drive yourself crazy with scanning through all the conditions, symptoms, and cures you can find online today. Sometimes it takes research and experience to find answers. Sometimes there isn't an answer.

But today, we are rewarded with endless **answers** without any research time or commitment. We think we are living in a time where we are more connected and educated than ever when in all actuality, we are disconnected and misinformed on more matters than not.

Sometimes there isn't a concrete answer that can be so easily comparable to the situation someone you follow is facing. Most things are **circumstantial and unique** and, in a world where everyone's starting to act more and more alike, this can really blur the lines.

Not utilizing all areas of our brain and not thinking for ourselves diminishes personal power while allocating that power to others. We are more than the opinion or judgment of others. We are who we are. You are you.

Create your own boundaries and be honest with yourself. **The only reassurance you need is from yourself.**

We've reached a point where we need more unique authentic expression, organic creation that can only come for you. Form thoughts that are truly yours. Steer away from the negative and ugly energy that pollutes the digital airspace. No longer emulate what someone else is doing, but allow yourself to experience what's happening on your own personal path.

We all have intuition. Our gut always knows the answer; however, we don't always choose to listen to it. But choosing to listen to your most natural instincts helps as you live out your truth. Being in touch with this side of yourself will build strength while guiding you in a positive direction.

I hope to encourage you to not only think for yourself but just be yourself. Follow and express yourself in healthy ways. Be kind to yourself and be kind to those around you. Act with sincerity, love with passion and communicate organically. **We have no time to waste.** And now, more than ever, **we need you.**

About The Author

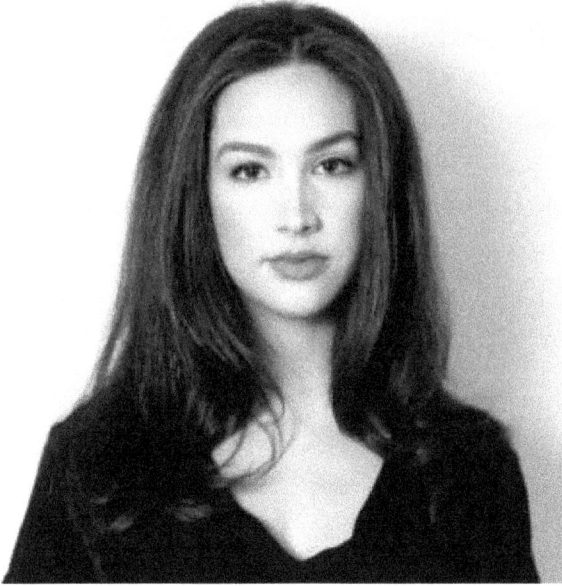

Headshot Credit: Can Ahtam

Alyssa Lynn Malmquist was born in Worcester, Massachusetts. Early on she acquired the label of bold. She always considered herself a creative, expressing herself through theater, fashion, web design, social media, and, eventually her most powerful form of expression, writing. After graduating college with a Bachelor of Science degree in Business Marketing, Alyssa moved to South Boston as she was pushed into corporate life for the next three years. She didn't adapt well. She loved her city life outside of work but still felt she wasn't reaching her fullest potential. Alyssa craved so much more. So at the age of 25, she quit her job in digital marketing and decided to drive cross-country to pursue writing and acting in Los Angeles. She left the greatest friends, the most supportive family, and all she had ever known in Massachusetts, so she could see what she was made of on her own. One year in Los Angeles pushed Alyssa to work on many projects, including the completion of her first book, *Put the Damn Phone Down.*

Instagram @alyssalynnmalmquist
Facebook facebook.com/alyssalynnmalmquist
Website alyssamalmquist.com

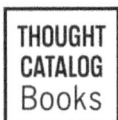

THOUGHT
CATALOG
Books

Thought Catalog Books is a publishing house owned by The Thought & Expression Company, an independent media group based in Brooklyn, NY. Founded in 2010, we are committed to facilitating thought and expression. We exist to help people become better communicators and listeners in order to engender a more exciting, attentive, and imaginative world.

Visit us on the web at
www.thoughtcatalogbooks.com and *www.collective.world*.

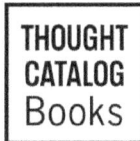

www.ingramcontent.com/pod-product-compliance
Lightning Source LLC
Chambersburg PA
CBHW032120280326
41933CB00009B/927